PREF[ACE]

Defects and diseases of th[e] [eye are on the] increase in recent times.

An observation of kindergarten and primary school students immediately confirms the truth in the above statement. A large number of young children can be seen wearing spectacles. Among these, there are some whose vision is not improved much even by glasses. The reasons for such problems and their solutions need to be found.

Today, the layman is more conscious than ever before about his ocular health. Many people ask what should be done to keep the eyes in good condition and what precautions they should take to prevent ocular defects in their children. This book is meant for such persons.

I have faith that one who follows the suggestions and methods given in this book will succeed in maintaining one's ocular health and keep at bay eye-problems.

At the same time, the general health also needs consideration. To have healthy eyes, a healthy body is essential. The food we eat has an effect on our health and the eyes. Hence a separate chapter on diet has been included.

The methods of preserving ocular health given in this book are extremely simple and easy to practise. They would consume a minimum of time. Assimilation of these methods in the daily routine will prove worthwhile.

Prevention is always better than cure. This book deals with prevention of eye defects and diseases. For treatment of existing ocular defects or diseases, a separate book is being prepared.

Opinions and suggestions will be gratefully accepted.

– **Authors**

CONTENTS

Published by Navneet Publications (India) Ltd., Dantali, Gujarat.
Printed by Sagar Offset, Ahmedabad. Tel. 2660 0622

[3 – 8 – 2006 (15) : 4]

1. INTRODUCTION

Of all the sense organs, the eye is most vital. Without sight, all the worldly gains and material achievements are of little use; the life becomes burdensome and meaningless. Eyes are invaluable.

Yet, what do we do to keep our eyes healthy and to maintain good vision? We do almost nothing. Most of us do not even realise that something can be done for the eyes. Indeed, we have entrusted the work of eye-care to the Almighty. If at all something wrong happens to our eyes or sight, we curse the fate, little realising that it is the result of our own carelessness and apathy.

We save for the rainy day. We insure our life against disasters. We ceaselessly try to obtain a good house to live in. But we do nothing to procure a good body, in which God resides. We cannot hope for good eyes without good health. 'Good eyes in a good body' is an apt idiom.

The advent of modern civilisation has necessitated the exaction of various types of work from our eyes. The eyes are excessively taxed. Our reading and writing activities continue unabated even during the late hours. Such incessant reading or writing deprives the eyes of their legitimate rest and relaxation. It strains our delicate eyes.

Advertisements have led some people to resort to the use of certain eye-drops or ointments. But it would be too much to expect anything really worthwhile of such drops. We should pay attention to the correct ways of using our eyes and develop such habits as would maintain the eye-health.

It is true that eyes are meant for seeing. But their excessive use must be stopped. At the same time, we should learn the methods to keep eyes and the body strong and healthy. Without good health, one cannot hope for good eyes.

Remember that roots of eye-troubles like cataract, glaucoma, retinal diseases, etc. are found in ill-health. If one wants to stay away from such troubles, one should care for one's body. Good health depends upon the right diet and vigorous exercise. One should continuously strive to maintain the powers of the digestive system at peak level. If the body along with the eyes is cared for, one can hope of perfect sight even in old age.

2. CAUSES OF VISUAL TROUBLES

All the causes for defective eye-sight are yet to be found out. However, some factors are known to be responsible. They have been enlisted below. One or more of these factors might be responsible for a particular eye-defect.

(1) **Hereditory causes :** The role of heredity in visual defects is still controversial. Many a times, visual defects are found to be present even at birth. Such defects include high myopia (pathological variety), high astigmatism, keratoconus, etc. Normally, a child at birth has 2.50 diopters of hypermetropia. Hypermetropia of a greater magnitude should also be considered abnormal.

It is true that if both the parents have good eye-sight, their children rarely suffer from visual defects. If both the parents have similar visual defects e.g. high myopia, a similar defect in their children is found much oftener. That is why such couples are advised against marrying each other.

(2) **Acquired causes :**

(a) **Eye-strain :** According to the prevalent belief, visual defects lead to eye-strain. However, there are experts who believe that eye-strain is not the result but the cause of visual defects.

Incorrect or excessive use of the eyes or inadequate rest to the eyes gives rise to eye-strain. Besides, since the eyes and the mind are intimately connected, mental tension may also give rise to eye-strain.

(b) **Excessive close work :** This factor has a major share in creating or increasing eye-defects like myopia. It is an indisputable fact that eyes are meant to look at distant objects. Yet, today eyes are forced to do excessive and continuous close work. The cases of short-sightedness increase with the increase in education.

The present system of education plays a major role in creating eye troubles. An average child is forced to become a book-worm. Besides studying the texts, a student has to indulge in extra-curricular reading, home-work, etc. Thus, day in and day out, he has to engage his eyes in close work.

It has been observed that children studying through English medium more often suffer from defective vision. English, after all, is a foreign language. Compared to our own languages, it is quite difficult to learn. Consequently, education through English medium means a lot of hard work and concentration on the part of students. Mental strain arising out of such education leads to eye-strain and finally to eye-defects.

The eyes are not fully developed at birth. Normally, they continue to develop till the child is of six years. Education starts much earlier, usually when a child is $2\frac{1}{2}$ to 3 years old. In other words, under-developed and delicate eyes are subjected to unwanted and unaccustomed burden of close work. It would not be an exaggeration to say that we educate our children at the cost of their sight.

It is observed that the body and a visual defect develop simultaneously. So the progress of a visual defect in a person usually gets arrested by the time he reaches an age of about twenty years, when the physical growth is almost complete. In the past it was found that children experienced difficulty in seeing at the age of about 13 – 14 years. The defect could not increase to a greater extent, as it did not have a great span to grow. But nowadays, unfortunately, we find that a visual defect starts in most children at the age of 5 – 6 years. Since the physical development of children is very quick, this visual defect also increases rapidly in a very short time; and when the body is fully developed, we observe that the defect has also developed to a great extent. It also happens nowadays that the defect continues to increase even after the completion of physical growth. This is an alarming situation.

Dr. Francis Young and Dr. Donald Harvis from America have conclusively proved that near-sightedness is directly related to close work.

This fact has also been proved under controlled conditions. Before the advent of education, the incidence of short-sightedness was negligible in Alaska. Under the regime of America, education was made compulsory. In a short span of 10 years, almost 75% of the Alaskan children had developed short-sightedness. It will be interesting to note that in tribals who still solely rely upon hunting or farming for their livelihood, short-sightedness is rare.

Watching television or video should also be termed close work for all practical purposes. This factor is more important for urban youngsters. Indeed, this is one more reason why parents should be on their alert for their children's eye-care.

(c) **Unnecessary use of glasses :** It has been mentioned earlier that eyes continuously undergo changes in their shape. During the day, the keenness of sight varies. Under favourable conditions, the sight is sharper and vice-versa. When a person uses glasses for a particular eye-defect, he makes that defect permanent.

According to a survey, the degree of myopia decreases during the vacation owing to lack of close work. At the end of the vacation, the vision is seen to be much improved. A student who continuously uses glasses during the vacation (because he is advised to do so!) denies the eyes the chance for self-improvement.

If the visual defect is not correctly estimated or if glasses are not made precisely to the prescription, eye-strain might be caused, which would worsen the existing eye-defect or create a new one.

(3) **Pathological causes :** Certain eye diseases or defects also lead to defects of vision. Though this subject is beyond the scope of this book, a mention of such conditions would be worthwhile.

Displacement of the eye-lens may give rise to visual defects. Its forward displacement gives rise to myopia (short-sightedness), backward displacement causes hyper-metropia (long-sightedness) and oblique displacement causes astigmatism (irregular sight). The removal of cataractous eye-lens also causes high hypermetropia. A tumour at the rear part of the eyeball may also cause hypermetropia. Congenital glaucoma leads to progressive lengthening of the eyeball and hence myopia. An increase in the refractive index (density) of eye-lens causes myopia. Defects of the cornea give rise to astigmatism. Such defects include corneal injuries or incisions (surgical) and keratoconus (cone-shaped cornea).

Most of the above mentioned conditions call for surgery. Defects of cornea can sometimes be controlled by contact lenses.

(4) **Metabolic causes :** Cataract and Glaucoma are the chief causes of visual defects in old age. Both these diseases are, to a greater or lesser extent, the results of improper metabolism. Excessive use of milk, milk products, tea, coffee, alcohol combined with defeciencies of vitamins gives rise to these diseases.

If one considers the above facts, it becomes clear that to avoid visual troubles, one should : (1) prevent eye-strain,

(2) curtail close work, (3) try to get rid of existing errors of refraction (i.e., eye-numbers), (4) develop such dietary habits that would benefit the eyes, (5) try to maintain peak general health.

3. DIET

Good health and good sight go hand in hand. Without good health, one cannot hope for good sight, especially in old age. Eyes are a part of the body. Any treatment of eye troubles ignoring general health is not likely to succeed fully.

To maintain or to improve health, we should cultivate correct dietary habits. To keep the digestive system efficient, we should eat at the same time every day, we should fast occasionally and should exercise regularly.

With advancing age, the efficiency of digestive organs ebbs. At 40–45 years of age, if we continue to eat all those things which we ate in youth, we may not be able to digest them completely. Imperfect metabolism is probably one of the reasons for old-age eye-problems. Hence after middle age our diet should be one which is simple and easily digestible.

One who wishes to maintain perfect eye-sight even in old age should make a firm resolution to cut down the intake of sweet, fried or spicy things, very cold eatables, tea, coffee and alcoholic beverages. The diet should be simple, natural and nutritious. This would ensure good health and good eyes.

The total quantity of food eaten should also be taken into account. One should eat to live, and not live to eat, as is the case with most of us. Excessive food is a burden to the digestive organs and invariably leads to indigestion and other troubles. Many a physicians see digestive disorders at the root of all other diseases. In short, moderate quantity of well-balanced diet is beneficial to the body.

A well-balanced diet is one which comprises of :
1. Carbohydrates   – approximately   40 – 50 %
2. Proteins   – approximately   15 – 20 %
3. Fats   – approximately   3 – 5 %
4. Vitamins & Minerals – approximately   20 – 25 %
5. Fibres & roughage – approximately   5 – 7 %

Carbohydrates are easily available from cereals, pulses and edible roots like potatoes and sweet potatoes. It is desirable that a meal should have only one type of carbohydrates.

Milk, pulses, meat, fish and eggs are the chief sources of proteins. Though animal-proteins are easily digestible and complete, yet their use is undesirable because of the presence of an amino-acid methionine which is believed to damage the blood-vessels.

Fats can be obtained from ghee, butter and various oils.

Vitamins and minerals are found aplenty in various raw vegetables and fruits. Vitamins and minerals are of paramount importance for general as well as eye-health. Fruits and vegetables also supply us with fibres and roughage which are necessary for the movement of the bowels. Other sources of roughage are wheat-bran, whole pulses, whole cereals, etc.

The importance of various vitamins for the eyes and their availability has been discussed in the following paragraphs :

Vitamin A : The importance of vitamin A for the eyes is well-known. Deficiency of vitamin A results into dry eyes (xerosis) and night blindness. If the deficiency is not reversed in time, the anterior part of the eye i.e., cornea slowly softens and melts, ultimately leading to blindness. The early symptoms of vitamin A deficiency are red, dry (lustreless) and gritty eyes, easy fatiguability of the eyes and difficulty in seeing in dark.

The recommended daily dose of vitamin A is 5000 international units for adults and 2000 i. u. for children. In conditions of deficiency, high doses of vitamin A (2,00,000 i. u. to adults and 50,000 i. u. to children) can be given.

Natural sources of vitamin A include milk, butter, buttermilk, ghee, codliver oil, ripe mango, papaya, carrot, melon, date, fig, orange, cabbage, tomato, karela (bitter gourd) and all green leafy vegetables.

Vitamin B : Vitamin B, too, is necessary for good sight. It is in fact a group of vitamins chiefly comprising of vitamin B_1 (thiamine), B_2 (riboflavin), B_6 (pyridoxin) and B_{12} (cobalamine).

Deficiency of vitamin B results into swelling of the optic nerve (retro-bulbar neuritis). The early symptoms of vitamin B deficiency are painful and watery eyes and a burning sensation in the eyes.

The recommended daily dose of each of the members of vitamin B group is about 1 mg.

The natural sources of vitamin B include milk, curd, eggs, meat, bran (especially wheat-bran), soyabeans, apples, oranges, bananas, grapes, green peas, carrots, cucumber, pumpkin, karela (bitter gourd), raddish, cabbage, green coconut, almond, groundnut and pulses.

Vitamin C : Vitamin C is also essential to the eyes. It gives strength to the blood vessels.

Its deficiency results into tired, heavy eyes and occassional bleeding in the conjunctiva.

Recommended daily dose of vitamin C is 80 mg. for adults and 30–50 mg. for children.

Natural sources of vitamin C include all sweet-sour fruits. Amla, lemon, orange, sweet lemon (mosambi), guava, tomatoes, apple, pineapple, papaya, cabbage, etc. are good sources of vitamin C.

The best way of obtaining vitamin C is to take a glass of water having juice of one lemon in it, early in the morning. If amlas are available, it is preferable to take two-three

Prevention is better than cure

GALA

CARE OF THE EYES

A book for those who want to keep their
eyes and vision good throughout their life

by

Dr. Dhiren Gala

B.Sc., D.H.M.S., D.O., D.Ac.,
C.G.O., C.C.H., A.R.S.H.

Recipient of a gold medal for extraordinary
work in the field of Alternative Therapeutics

With

Dr. D. R. Gala
N.D., D.N.O., D.C.O.

Dr. Sanjay Gala
M.B. (BOM.), M.S. (ENT)

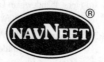

NAVNEET PUBLICATIONS (INDIA) LIMITED

Navneet House, Gurukul Road, Memnagar, Ahmadabad–380 052. Phone : 6630 5000	**Navneet Bhavan,** B. S. Road, Dadar, Mumbai–400 028. Phone : 6662 6565

DHANLAL BROTHERS DISTRIBUTORS

70, Princess Street, Mumbai–400 002.
Phone : 2201 7027

G 4503

Visit us at : www.navneet.com | e-mail : npil@navneet.com **Price : Rs. 18.00**

Dr. Dhiren Gala

1st Floor, Abbas Building 'A',
Near Tilak Market, Jalbhai Lane, Harkishandas Hospital Road,
Grant Road (East), Mumbai – 400 004. Phone : 2386 7275
Timings : 4 to 7 p. m.

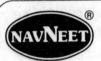 **NAVNEET PUBLICATIONS (INDIA) LIMITED**

Mumbai : 1. Bhavani Shankar Road, Dadar, **Mumbai – 400 028.**
(Tel. 6662 6565 • Fax : 6662 6352)

2. **Navyug Distributors :** Road No. 8, M. I. D. C., Next to Indian Institute of Packaging, Marol, Andheri (East), **Mumbai – 400 093.** (Tel. 2821 4186 • Fax : 2835 2758)

Ahmadabad : Navneet House, Gurukul Road, Memnagar, **Ahmadabad – 380 052.**
(Tel. 6630 5000)

Bangalore : Sri Balaji's, No. 12, 2nd Floor, 3rd Cross, Malleswaram,
Bangalore – 560 003. (Tel. 2346 5740)

Bhopal : Navneet Sadan, E-7/728, Arera Colony, Shahpura, **Bhopal – 462 016.** (Tel. 427 8544)

Chennai : 30, Sriram Nagar, North Street, Alwarpet, **Chennai – 600 018.** (Tel. 2434 6404)

Delhi : 2-E/23, Orion Plaza, 2nd & 3rd Floor, Jhandewalan Extn.,
New Delhi – 110 055. (Tel. 2361 0170)

Hyderabad : Kalki Plaza, Plot No. 67, Krishna puri Colony, West Maredpalley,
Secunderabad – 500 026. (Tel. 2780 0146)

Kolkata : Newar Bhavan, 1st Floor, No. 87, Chowringhee Road, **Kolkata – 700 020.**
(Tel. 2223 2497)

Nagpur : 63, Opp. Shivaji Science College, Congress Nagar, **Nagpur – 440 012.** (Tel. 242 1522)

Nashik : Dharmaraj Plaza, Old Gangapur Naka, Gangapur Road,
Nashik – 422 005. (Tel. 231 0627)

Navsari : 3/C, Arvind Nagar Society, Lunsikui Road, **Navsari – 396 445.** (Tel. 244 186)

Patna : 1st Floor, 36-D, Sahdeo Mahto Marg, Srikrishnapuri, **Patna – 800 001.** (Tel. 220 4921)

Pune : Navneet Bhavan, 1302, Shukrawar Peth, Near Sanas Plaza, Bajirao Road, **Pune – 411 002.**
(Tel. 2443 1007)

Surat : 1, Ground Floor, Sri Vallabh Complex, Kotwal Street, Nanpara,
Surat – 395 001. (Tel. 246 3927)

Vadodara : F-1, Vaidya Vatika, Opp. Hanuman Wadi, Sardar Bhuvan Khancho,
Vadodara – 390 001.

tablespoons of amla juice mixed with a glassful of water early in the morning.

Vitamin D : Cases of cataract have been reported due to vitamin D deficiency. Thus vitamin D is also necessary for healthy eyes.

The recommended daily dose of vitamin D is 400 i.u.

Natural sources of vitamin D inculde milk, butter, eggs, liver, cod-liver oil, etc. The best source of vitamin D is sun. One should take direct sun-rays over the body for at least 15 minutes every day.

4. PHYSICAL EXERCISE

Exercise is as essential as a nourishing diet for the maintenance of good health. One should perform yoga and other exercises because they definitely stimulate the functioning of the digestive system, regulate and activate the process of metabolism and enable the body to resist disease.

It is necessary that one should learn yoga and other exercises from an expert and experienced person and then perform them carefully and regularly. Everyone should possess two or three books on yoga and other exercises. The elders should explain the necessity of exercises to all the members of the family. Yoga exercises are undoubtedly beneficial to physical health and mental health as well. Yoga exercises are not only good for physical health but also give true mental peace.

Yoga exercises are congenial to all persons irrespective of their age or sex. Besides, they can play an important role in curing many diseases. Yoga exercises cost neither money nor much time and do not require any equipment or contrivance. No big space is necessary to perform these exercises. They rarely cause fatigue or uneasiness. Health achieved by such exercises, not involving spasmodic movements, gives unrivalled happiness.

Deep breathing, Udiyan, Vaksha-vikas, Chakrasana, Parshwa-chakrasana, Yoga-mudra, Paschimottanasana, Halasana, Supta-vajrasana, Sarvangasana, Pet-chalan, Utthita – dwipadasana, Shirshasana, etc., are among the main yoga exercises. Shirshasana is considered to be useful for keeping the eyes healthy, since it improves their blood circulation.

Before starting the exercises, it would be preferable to drink a glass of water kept overnight in a copper vessel. Some lemon juice may be added to the water after transferring it from the copper vessel to a drinking glass, provided the person does not suffer from joint-disorders. In the winter season, amla should be preferred to lemon juice. Even those suffering from joint-disorders can take amla juice.

Eye exercises should be added to the general exercises with a view to keeping the eyes healthy. We find that most persons do not include the eye exercises in their routine exercises. The eye exercises are equally necessary. The following chapters describe the exercises meant specially for the eyes.

A practice of Shavasana at the end of exercises is always beneficial. Shavasana should be performed for ten minutes twice a day : in the morning (after exercises) and at night before going to bed. It is necessary for the health of the body and the mind.

The method of practising Shavasana * : Lie down straight on your back without a pillow beneath the head. Keep your arms extended and parallel to your body. Relax all the parts of your body. Slow down the breathing rhythm. Close the eyes and concentrate upon the tip of your nose as if to see the nose with eyes closed. Relax your body to the condition as a corpse. Pray silently to your favourite god. If

---

* According to various texts on Yoga, while practising Shavasana, the mind is to be kept blank, not allowing any thoughts to enter it. But this is not quite possible for everybody. Hence the method described above deviates slightly from the standard method in that it advises the recitation of 'mantras'.

you like to recite 'mantras' during Shavasana, count those 'mantras' silently on the tips of your finger for ten minutes (predetermine the number of the 'mantras' necessary to complete ten minutes); or, if possible, keep an alarm clock which rings at a fixed time. This will be most appropriate. Forget everything while silently chanting 'mantras'. Tell the members of your family not to disturb you while you are practising Shavasana.

Practising Shavasana in this way gives mental rest which in turn gives rest to the eyes. The peace of mind keeps your eyes free from strain. Also, try constantly to keep your temperament as cool as possible.

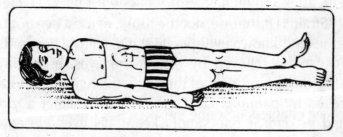

Shavasana

5. TEN GOOD HABITS FOR KEEPING EYES IN GOOD CONDITION

Just as general health can be preserved by doing physical exercises, ocular health can be maintained by certain good habits. The ten good habits described below help to maintain good eyesight. As these activities become regular habits in due course of time, no extra time is required to be spared for them.

(1) **Water-Splash :** Splash cold water over the closed eyes three or four times a day. Ice-water or water from a refrigerator will also serve the purpose. Splash water over the eyes while washing the face in the morning, before taking the meals and at bed-time.

Method : Fill the mouth with as much water as it can contain. Keeping the mouth full of water splash water over the closed eyes eight to ten times from a distance of four to five inches. If possible, do not wipe the water on the face. Let it dry of its own. Empty the mouth now.

(2) Palming : Palming means covering the closed eyes with the palms. When the eyes are fatigued or exhausted, they can be relaxed by palming. A five-minute palming twice or thrice a day is a must. Count upto eight hundred for a five-minute palming. Alternately, listen to two records of music or songs, each of three minutes. The purpose is well served while listening to slow melodious music.

"Strain is the cause, not the result, of most eye troubles," says the well-known eye-specialist, Dr. Harold Peppard. This strain can be relieved by resting the eyes, especially the sensitive innermost coat of the eye – 'the retina'. This can be achieved by palming. One can still tell whether a room is lighted or dark if one simply keeps his eyes closed. This means that light is entering his eyes. This can be prevented by covering the closed eyes with palms. Complete rest is necessary to preserve good eyesight. The eyes, while being palmed, experience pitchy darkness which gives them good rest.

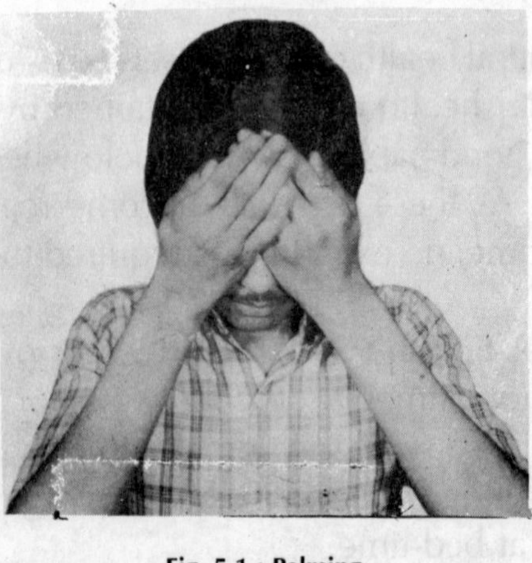

Fig. 5.1 : Palming

Method : Palming has been found to be most efficacious and should be cultivated as a daily habit by all. In palming, the closed eyes are covered with the palms of hands (both the palms slightly cupped, the fingers being crossed on the fore-head) in such a way as to avoid pressure or touching on the eye-balls. Take care that the outside light does not reach the eyes. Imagine perfect darkness before the eyes and then meditate.

Method of Palming – 1 : Sit on a chair in front of a table. Place the elbows on the table and do palming as shown in the figure.

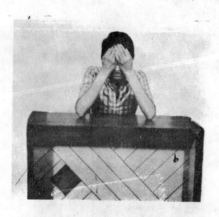

Fig. 5.2 : Palming in front of a table

Method of Palming – 2 : Sit on the ground or on a cot, the back touching the wall. Raise the knees to the chest. Rest the head on the wall. Put the elbows on the knees and practise palming as shown in the figure. This is the best and most comfortable method.

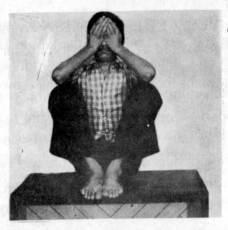

Fig. 5.3 : Palming on the ground or on a cot

Method of Palming – 3 : Sit on a chair. Put a small pillow on the thighs. Support the elbow on the pillow and do palming as shown in the figure. This method also is convenient.

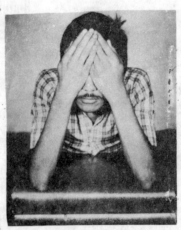

Fig. 5.4 : Palming with the help of a pillow

If, after the water-splash, palming with wet hands and wet face is performed, the eyes get coolness in addition to the advantage of the palming.

(3) Washing the feet with cold water : The feet should be washed with cold water twice a day and at night before going to bed. Rub the feet on the wet tiles of the bath-room for two or three minutes. Pour cold water on the feet while rubbing them on the tiles. This practice induces sound sleep which in turn helps to maintain good eyesight.

Massaging the bottoms of the feet with cow's ghee or pure castor oil seems to serve the same purpose; that is, to have a good effect on the eyes through the feet.

(4) Eye-bath : Bathe the eyes with cold water or Triphala water or weak saline (salt water) once or twice a day.

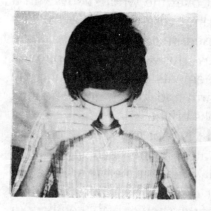
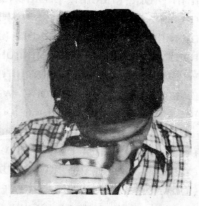

Fig. 5.5 : Eye-wash with eye cups	Fig. 5.6 : Eye-wash with a small bowl

Fill the eye-wash cups with water up to their brims. Keep the eye-wash cups straight, bend the head and dip the eyes in the water. Blink gently in the water. The eyes can be washed in a small bowl also. Wash the eyes for about a minute.

(5) Sun-rays : Sun-rays are very beneficial to the eyes. Let the eyes be exposed to the tender rays of the sun in the early morning and at sunset. When the sun is bright, close your eyes and face the sun.

Method : Sit or stand comfortably facing the sun with eyes closed. Then slowly turn the head to the left and then to the right. Repeat this exercise fifty times on each side. After enjoying the sun, splash the eyes with cold water and do palming for at least five minutes.

(6) **Moonlight :** In the moonlit nights, whenever possible, lie down on back facing the sky. Blink while looking at the moon. Keep the eyes relaxed. Practise this for ten to fifteen minutes. Blinking at the moon is beneficial to the eyes.

(7) **Eye-steam :** Once a week bathe the closed eyes with the steam of salted water. Fill in a big bowl with the boiling salt-water. Put the bowl on the ground. Sit in front of it in prone-kneeling position. Cover the whole body with a quilt or a blanket and take steam over the closed eyes. This method is similar to the one used in cold and coughs. Take the steam for about five minutes. This will cause perspiration which removes the harmful elements collected around the eyes. Eye muscles become warm and loosen up, benefiting the eyes. Besides, the face looks bright.

(8) **Shower on the head :** Except for some imperative necessity, do not pour hot water on the head in ordinary circumstances. After taking the bath and before wiping the body, take cold water shower on your head for about two minutes. If there is no facility of the shower bath, gently pour cold water from a jug on your head. This must be done slowly. Take at least half a minute to pour the jugful of water on the head. Then wipe the body. It is advantageous to do this as a regular habit.

(9) **Clay on the eyes :** Take clay of any colour (preferably black). It should be sifted and without grits. It should be obtained from the surroundings of a pond or from the virgin ground. It should be free from chemical fertilizers.

Method : Moisten clay with cold water and make round, flat and small lumps from it. Put these lumps on the closed eyes for about ten minutes. Cover the lumps with a dry piece of cloth. Clay has the virtue of drawing out poison. It gives coolness and strength also. It should not be kept on the eyes for more than ten minutes.

(10) Facial massage : For a minute or two every day, vigorously massage the skin of the face and the neck with a napkin soaked in cold water. Occasionally use hot and cold napkins alternately. Start with a hot nepkin; massage the face for a minute; then take a cold napkin and massage the face for half a minute. Repeat this process three-four times. This method refreshes the eyes and improves the blood-circulation of the face.

* * * * *

Various methods of relaxing and refreshing the eyes have been discussed in the preceding paragraphs. However, it is not necessary to follow all these methods every day. Water-splashing, eye-wash and palming being more important should be done every day. Others can be done twice or thrice a week, as and when time permits.

6. CORRECT USE OF EYES

A normal, healthy eye can see distant as well as near objects clearly, without any strain. A person with subnormal vision may see distant objects blurred. He makes an effort to see which becomes obvious by his squeezing the eye-lids. This should be avoided as it causes strain to the eyes. A similar strain is produced when one stares at a particular object. A normal eye is continuously moving. It changes its focus rapidly as it views one place and then another. On the other hand, an abnormal eye remains more or less steady as can be seen in the cases of high myopia. Thus, it is desirable to keep the eyes constantly moving. Instead of viewing the whole of a large object at the same time, focus the attention on small parts of that object. Move the sight over its outlines. At the same time keep the eyes relaxed.

It would be worthwhile to know and learn how the eyes should be used while reading, writing, sewing, knitting, watching T. V. or cinema, etc.

(1) **Blinks :** Learn to blink frequently. Initially this may have to be done consciously. Later it becomes a habit. While reading, blink at least twice while completing a whole line. Blinking rests the eyes. Blinking can never be an obstacle in work since the eye-lids hardly touch each other.

(2) **Reading and writing :** While reading or writing, never hold the book too close to the eyes. A distance of at least 12 inches is desirable.

After reading for about an hour continuously, it is necessary to rest the eyes. This can be accomplished by keeping the eyes lightly closed for a short period or by splashing cold water over the eyes. However, the best way is palming.

(3) **Reading in moving vehicles :** Reading should be kept to minimum while travelling in a jerky, fast-moving vehicle. If at all one reads, he should frequently shift the sight out through the window and observe outer objects moving backwards. This would give the eyes some rest and keep them relaxed.

(4) **Reading at night :** Do not read in dazzling or excessively bright light. While reading with the help of a table-lamp, see that the light does not fall directly on the book. It should fall a little away from the book. Similarly, do not strain your eyes by reading in very dim light. Florescent light is better than the light from electric bulbs.

High voltage electric bulbs or mercury lamps in large shops which dazzle the eyes are harmful to the eyesight. Never stare at them.

(5) **Cinema – T. V. :** Viewing of cinema or T. V. should be curtailed. Children below the age of 12 years should not be allowed to see them often since it is during this period that there is the greatest possibility of the development of some ocular defect. The eye-defects of the children can generally be prevented, provided the children are properly taken care of. The children should be educated not to indulge in habits like long T. V. sessions which cause strain to their eyes. Repeating such sessions day in and day out is even more harmful.

While viewing the cinema or T. V. sit comfortably with the head slightly inclined backward. Raise the chin so that the upper lid remains half-closed. Do not forget to blink frequently. Do not lean forward to see. Keep the eyes relaxed and moving.

(6) **Sewing and knitting :** While engaged in sewing or knitting, shift the sight with the movement of the needle. Shift the sight and do not keep it fixed at any particular place on the cloth.

(7) **Goggles :** It is not undesirable to wear good-quality goggles in strong sunlight. Excessive heat and dazzling light of the sun contributes towards eye-strain and may damage the eyes. One should use goggles of high quality only.

However, the constant and continuous use of goggles is certainly harmful to the eyes. Natural light is essential and beneficial to the eyes. Wearing goggles day and night weakens the eyes. Besides, their power of resistance decreases. Weak eyes become the victims of many diseases. Such eyes become photophobic (abnormally sensitive to light), lose their natural lustre and become dry.

7. EXERCISES FOR STRENGTHENING EYES

This chapter covers only a few exercises which are helpful in preserving good eyesight. The eye exercises described below should be done regularly and sincerely. One who does other general exercises should add these eye exercises to one's daily routine.

(1) Eye-pressing and Sinhamudra

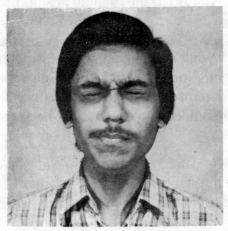

Fig. 7.1 : Eye-pressing

Eye-pressing : As shown in the figure, firmly shut both the eye-lids so as to bring about a squeezing effect on the eyes. Maintain this pressure and count twelve. Then relax the eye-lids. Rest the eyes for a short while by keeping them lightly closed. Then start the next part of this exercise i.e., sinhamudra.

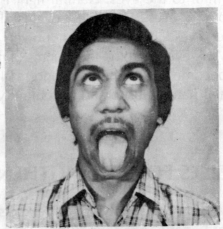

Fig. 7.2 : Sinhamudra

Sinhámudra (Lion pose) : Open the mouth as wide as possible. Bring the tongue out as much as possible as shown in the figure. Then look at the ceiling without raising the head or straining the eyes. Maintain this position and count twelve slowly. Then return to the original position. Rest the eyes for a short while by keeping them closed.

For the first two days repeat the above two exercises alternately, three times each. Then for the next two days repeat them four times and then five times. Do not increase the number of repetitions to more than five times. After completing the above exercises perform a hundred-count palming. Then begin the second group of exercises.

(2) Movements of the eyes to different directions : In performing the below-given exercises, the head should be kept steady. Only the eyes are to be moved. There are five different sets of exercises. After the completion of one set of the exercises, take rest for twenty counts before performing the next set of the exercises.

(A) Moving the eyes sidewards : This exercise consists of turning the eyes towards right and left, while keeping the head steady. Turn the eyes towards the right as much as possible without causing undue strain. Now blink once and turn the eyes towards the left as much as possible. Again blink and turn the eyes towards the right. Repeat twelve times (6 right side, 6 left side). Now rest the eyes by keeping them lightly closed and counting twenty. Then gently open the eyes and start the second set of exercises.

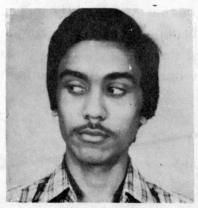

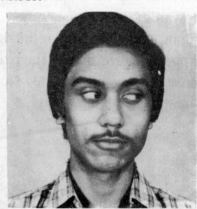

Fig. 7.3 : To the right side   **Fig. 7.4 : To the left side**

(B) Moving the eyes upward and downward : Keeping the head steady look up as much as possible. Now blink once and look down as much as possible. Again blink and look up. Repeat twelve times. Then rest the eyes by keeping them lightly closed and counting twenty.

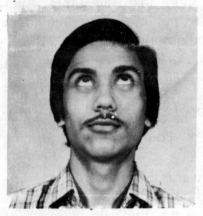 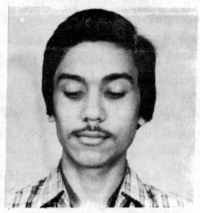

Fig. 7.5 : Upward   **Fig. 7.6 : Downward**

Now open the eyes and perform the next set of exercises.

(C) Moving the eyes to the right corner upward and to the left corner downward : Keeping the head steady look towards the right upper corner. Now blink once and look towards the left lower corner. Thus the eyes should be moved along a diagonal joining the right upper and left lower corner. Repeat twelve times. Then rest the eyes by keeping them closed for twenty counts. Now open the eyes and perform the next set of exercises.

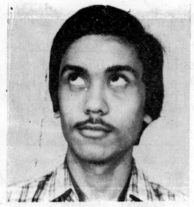

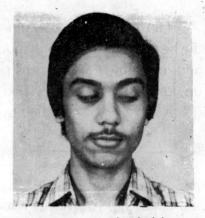

Fig. 7.7 : Upward to the right   Fig. 7.8 : Downward to the left

(D) Moving the eyes upward to the left and downward to the right : This exercise is similar to the set C exercise except that eyes should be moved along a diagonal joining the left upper corner and right lower corner as shown in the above figures. Again rest the eyes for twenty counts and start the next set of exercises.

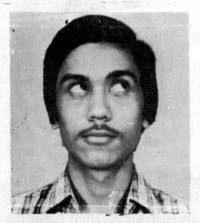

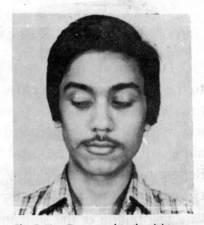

Fig. 7.9 : Upward to the left   Fig. 7.10 : Downward to the right

(E) Circular movements of the eyes : This exercise is a combination of the previous four sets of exercises. Keeping the head steady, move the eyes in circles with the help of the index finger. Looking continuously at the tip of the index finger, move the hand in circles around the face. Complete three clockwise circles. Then complete three anticlockwise circles. In similar fashion complete three – three more circles either way.

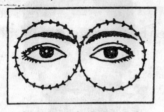
Fig. 7.11 : Clockwise circles

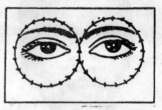
Fig. 7.12 : Anticlockwise circles

Note : For the first two days limit the number of repetitions to twelve. Increase the number of repetitions to sixteen for the next two days. Then continue with twenty repetitions (not more). After completing all the five sets of exercises, perform a hundred-count palming.

(3) Neck movements :

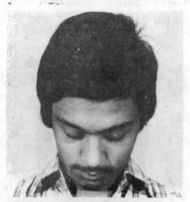
Fig. 7.13 : Head forward

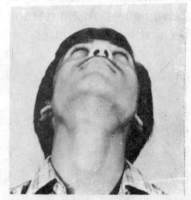
Fig. 7.14 : Head backward

(A) Bending the head forward and backward : At first bend the head forward. Press the chin to the throat. Look at the first button of the shirt for three counts. Then bend the head backwards as much as possible and look behind for three counts. Repeat this exercise twelve times, 6 – 6 times each side. Take rest for twenty counts and perform the following exercises.

(B) Right and left turning of the head : Turn the head to the right as much as possible. Look backwards as far as possible. Wait for three counts. Then gently turn the head to the left. Look backwards as far as possible. Wait for three counts. Repeat this exercise twelve times, 6 – 6 times each side. Rest for twenty counts and then begin the following third exercise.

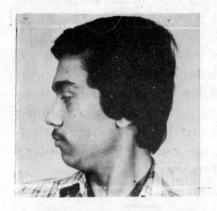 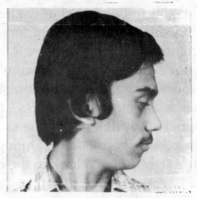

Fig. 7.15 : Head to the right side   Fig. 7.16 : Head to the left side

(C) Bending the head to the right and left shoulders : Bend the head towards the right shoulder. Look at the ceiling above for three counts. Then shift the sight downwards towards the floor near the foot and count up to three. Then bend the head towards the left shoulder and look at the

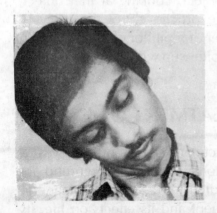 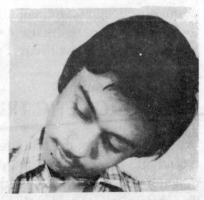

Fig. 7.17 : Head towards the right shoulder   Fig. 7.18 : Head towards the left shoulder

ceiling above for three counts. Without changing the position of the head look downwards for three counts. Repeat this exercise twelve times. Then take rest for twenty counts and begin the next exercise.

(D) **Rotating the head** : This exercise is a combination of the three exercises described above. In this exercise, the head is to be moved in circles. Start with the head bent fully forward. Keeping it bent forward, turn it so as to reach the right shoulder. From there, take the head fully backward and move it in an arc to reach the left shoulder. From there, bend it forward again, to reach the starting position. Complete three such anticlockwise circles. Then move the head in three clockwise circles in similar fashion. Thus altogether move the head in twelve circles. During this exercise keep on shifting the sight so as to look in the direction of the head.

After completing these exercises perform a hundred-count palming.

Note : Perform these exercises sixteen times after two days. Increase the repetitions to twenty (not more) after next two days.

(4) **Alternately looking at near and distant objects :** Hold your finger about an inch away from your nose tip. Look at the finger-tip and count three. Shift the gaze to a pre-determined very distant object. Looking at that object, count three again. Repeat the process thirty times. Every fourth day, increase the number of repititions by ten to reach a maximum number of sixty. Follow up with a hundred-count palming.

8. MAGNETIC TREATMENT OF EYES

Before discussing the effects of magnets on the eyes, it would be worthwhile to consider the background of magnetotherapy. Without taking into account, magneto-therapy's history, its development and its effects on life, its role in the treatment of eyes cannot be correctly understood.

As a scientific mode of treatment, magnetotherapy's evolution can be traced back to about fifty years. In America, Russia, Japan and some other developed countries, magneto-therapy has gained appreciable acceptance and popularity. In some other countries, it is spreading rapidly. In India, however, only a few know about magnetotherapy.

The early experiments with magnets were naturally performed on plants, insects and animals. These experiments brought to light some amazing facts. Dr. Medelin Barnothy of Illinois University, America has compiled a book 'Biological effects of magnetic field' which includes experimental findings of researchers from America, England, Russia, France, etc. It would be worthwhile to briefly consider some of these findings.

Seeds treated with magnets germinated earlier and grew faster. They showed a greater resistance to plant diseases and unfavourable weather. They grew into tall trees and bore heavy fruit. Seeds and plants irrigated with 'magnetised water' showed similar results.

Experiments were performed on a variety of animals including mice, rabbits and rhesus monkeys. When kept for a fixed period of time in a magnetic field for six weeks, these animals lived considerably longer. These animals could keep away degenerative changes of old age. Female rats experienced negligible difficulty at the time of delivering babies. Most important finding was remission of cancer. When animals suffering from cancer were continuously kept in a strong magnetic field, the cancer tumour shrunk in size and ultimately disappeared.

Effects of magnetic field on human beings : Every cell of our body is an electrical unit and hence possesses its own magnetic field. Therefore, it vibrates with a particular frequency.

The terminology of magnetotherapy defines disease as a condition in which there is a lack of harmony in the vibrations of cells of different organs. Whenever there is a disturbance in magnetic field of a tissue, its natural vibratory frequency is disrupted and disease ensues. Due to the altered vibratory frequency, that tissue or the organ cannot function co-ordinatedly with other organs, giving rise to a disease. If the natural frequency of vibration can be restored, disease can be overcome and health can be regained. Permanent magnets provide a steady magnetic field and help to restore health.

Direct beneficial effects of magnetic field : When magnets are kept in contact of a body-part, the later regains its natural frequency of vibration.

The electromagnetic waves emanating from the magnets penetrate deep into the body to reach each and every cell. The cell-material (cytoplasm) gets polarised. Polarisation imparts strength to the cells.

Magnetic field stimulates the growth of new cells, hastens wound-healing and encourages rapid union of broken bone. Magnetic field inhibits the activities of disease-causing micro-organisms and ultimately destroys them.

Indirect beneficial effects of magnetic field : All the body-fluids are affected by magnets. Many physical and chemical properties like density, viscosity, surface tension, etc. of fluilds undergo favourable changes.

Blood is also a body-fluid. The above mentioned effects are observed on blood too. Besides, the red blood corpuscles of the blood are affected due to the iron present in them.

When electromagnetic waves enter the blood-stream, eddy-currents are produced. These eddy-currents warm the blood and increase the number of ions present in blood.

When such ionised blood circulates in the body, benefits ensue. Deposits of cholesterol and calcium on the inner surface of blood-vessels are washed away. The slight increase in the blood's temperature regulates the various hormonal secretions. Warm blood helps to resolve swelling and decrease pain.

When our body is infected by disease-causing organisms, the number of white blood corpuscles increases; the erythrocyte sedimentation rate (E.S.R.) goes up. After appropriate treatment with magnets, the infection is overcome. The testimony to this fact is the decrease in the number of white blood corpuscles and the E.S.R.

In short, magnetised blood refreshes and rejuvenates the body-cells, improves the body's resistance to disease and increases the efficiency of various body-systems.

These are the indirect beneficial effects of magnetic field. Thus even when the magnets are applied to one part of the body, the whole body is affected and benefited.

Magnetised water : Physical and chemical properties of water are favourably affected by magnets. When magnetised water is drunk, it imparts health and vigour to the body. Digestion improves; gastric acidity decreases; the excretory system becomes more efficient. Magnetised water has been found to dissolve or disintegrate kidney or bladder stones.

Drinking water can be charged with magnetism by placing a glass/plastic bottle containing drinking water between attracting (i.e., north and south) poles of two strong magnets, overnight. This water should be consumed in doses of 100–125 ml., four times a day. This water may also be used to bathe eyes.

The effects of magnets on the eyes : Small, weak magnets can be used for local treatment of the eyes.

Most common eye ailments like burning, redness, itching, discharge (formation of mucous) and watering should be treated with south poles. Similarly, visual defects like short-sightedness and (myopic) astigmatism should be treated with south poles. On the other hand, visual defects like far-sightedness, (hypermetropic) astigmatism, presbyopia and eye-diseases like cataract, retinal degeneration and optic atrophy call for the north poles. For eye-treatment, a frame containing suitable magnets should be worn for 10–15 minutes, twice a day.

All the good effects of the magnetic field, discussed in the preceding paragraphs, take place on eyes too. It is the experience of the authors that regular use of magnets helps to prevent or cure many eye-diseases.

A person undertaking magnetic treatment of eyes should keep the following two points in mind :

(1) Cold water should not be splashed on the face or bath should not be taken for an hour before or after the magnetic treatment of the eyes.

(2) One should not worry if, during the first day or two of the treatment, the head feels slightly heavy.

Summary : Magnetotherapy is an effective yet harmless mode of treatment. The treatment of eyes with magnets has yielded very good results. Better results are obtained if along with the local treatment of the eyes, a generalised treatment of the whole body is also simultaneously undertaken. General health also depends upon right food and regular exercise. Treatment of eyes alone, disregarding other parts of the body is likely to succeed only partially. The various methods of applying magnets to improve general health or to get rid of diseases cannot be incorporated in this small book. The reader is advised to procure and study a few good books on magnetotherapy.

9. CARE OF CHILDREN'S EYESIGHT RIGHT FROM THEIR CHILDHOOD

It is a duty of parents to take care of their children's sight. If one or both of the parents suffer from visual defects, they should remain alert and take greater care of their children's eyesight. Such parents should prevent their children from excessively indulging in near works like reading, writing, drawing, painting, embroidering, etc. They should encourage their children to go out and play outdoor games. They should preferably educate their children through the medium of their mother-tongue which would entail lesser hard work on the part of their children. It is a known fact that the greater the burden of studies, the greater the mental tension and visual defects.

Children should be allowed only restricted viewing of television or video. Experiments have shown that a colour television does more harm to the eyes than a black and white television.

Parents should try to cultivate in their children the right habits for good sight and healthy eyes. Eye-wash, water-splashes and palming should be incorporated into daily schedule of activities. Children should be enlightened about the correct ways of using the eyes. They should not be allowed to read while lying down or to keep awake till late hours.

It is necessary that a child's eyes be tested before he joins a kindergarten. An eye-test should be repeated when the child is six years old. Thereafter a check-up every year is advisable.

Parents having visual defects themselves should remain more careful.

(1) Observe your child's reading–writing habits. Ensure that he reads or writes at a normal distance, like other children. If he insists on holding the print too close to his eyes, immediately get his eyes tested.

(2) If your child blinks more often than others, get his eyes tested.

(3) If your child is not able to recognise distant objects towards which you point, he might be suffering from short-sightedness (myopia). A child with short-sightedness partly shuts his eyes while seeing distant objects. His near vision is, however, good.

(4) If your child cannot recognise very small letters or dislikes close work, he might be suffering from long-sightedness (hypermetropia). People with such a defect may or may not have good distant vision.

(5) If your child does not look straight and tries to see by turning or tilting his head, he is likely to be suffering from some visual defect.

(6) If your child prefers to watch television or video from a very short distance, he might be suffering from defective eyesight. Normally he should be able to watch television with ease from a distance of 12 – 14 feet.

Vision passes through a process of development during the first six years of life. In other words, a child's vision is fully developed (6/9 or 6/6) by the time he is six years old. If at this time a child can see both near and distant objects clearly and with ease, his eyes can be considered normal.

You can test your child's sight yourself at home. The method of sight-testing is described in chapter ten.

If you test your child's sight every six months, any change in his eyesight can immediately be detected. Whenever necessary, it is advisable to consult an eye-specialist.

A thing that should be remembered is that small defects of sight can be overcome easily with appropriate eye-exercises. Such eye-exercises should be tried before going for spectacles.

10. EYESIGHT TESTING METHOD

It is worthwhile to keep three-four different eyesight testing charts in one's house. If the child is made to read a different chart every time, he is not likely to learn the letters by heart. After the completion of the test, the chart should be closed and kept out of the child's reach.

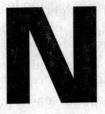

N

60 Metres

C T

36 M

O H E

24 M

L P A D

18 M

R T U L P

12 M

H N O A C F

9 M

D H P E X O L

6 M

A model of distant sight-testing chart

Let us study the distant vision testing chart with the help of the given model. In this chart, a big letter is printed on the top. Below the letter is the figure 60. The two letters smaller than the first one are below the figure 60. The figure 36 is printed below these two letters. Below the figure 36 there are three letters smaller than the above two letters and the figure 24 is printed below them. Similarly in the lines that follow, smaller and yet smaller letters are printed with the figures 18, 12, 9, 6, 5 & 4 respectively below them.

The figures in the chart indicate the distance at which these letters can be easily read by persons with normal eyesight. Thus the figure 60 indicates tnat a person with normal eyesight can read the letter above it from a distance of 60 metres. The letters with the figure 36 below them can be read by a normally-sighted person from a distance of 36 metres and so on. **For checking the eyesight, the distance should always be 6 metres.** If a person can read the letters of the seventh line comfortably from the distance of 6 metres, his vision is said to be normal. It is denoted as 6/6. Thus, eyesight is recorded as a fraction in which the numerator denotes the distance of the subject from the chart, which is usually 6 metres, and the denominator denotes the line which the subject reads. Thus 6/12 means that from 6 metres, a person can read only that line which a normally-sighted person would have read from the distance of 12 metres.

For testing distant vision, make use of the chart given at the end of this book. Record the vision of each eye separately, first without and then with glasses. See that the child does not strain his eyes whilst reading the letters on the chart.

The near vision should be tested with the help of the near vision testing chart given at the end of this book. The chart should be held 14 inches from the eyes and should be well-illuminated. A person with normal eyesight should be able to read even the smallest letters on the chart i.e., N_5.

The findings of near and distant vision testing should be noted down on a card as shown :

Name				Age		
Obsn. No.	Date		Right Eye		Left Eye	
			Without glasses	With glasses	Without glasses	With glasses
1		Distant vision				
		Near vision				
2						

The vision should be checked at regular intervals of time. This way, any change in vision can immediately be detected.

11. CONTACT LENSES

During the past few years, the demand for and the use of contact lenses have shown an unprecedented increase. It is necessary to enlighten people about some facts and fallacies regarding contact lenses.

The first contact lens came into existence in 1887. This lens was double-walled and was made of glass. The lens contained between its two walls, a substance called gelatin. At that time, however, there was no way of measuring the anterior curvature of the eye-ball. Hence the lens did not fit well on the eye and had to be discarded. In 1932, Dr. Joseph Dallos succeeded in measuring the curvature of the eye-ball and prepared a glass contact lens accordingly. This lens, however, happened to be too heavy to be worn comfortably even for a few seconds. In 1943, plastic contact lenses made their appearance. These lenses were made to fit on whole of the outer surface of the eye-ball and were termed scleral contact lenses. In 1948, corneal contact lenses came into

existence. Such lenses are fitted only on the transparent part
of the eye i.e., cornea.

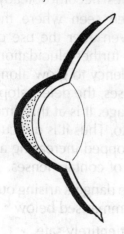

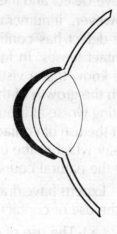

Fig. 11.1 : Scleral contact lens
(This lens is now obsolete.)

Fig. 11.2 : Corneal contact lens
(This lens is used widely nowadays.)

At present three types of corneal contact lenses are
available : hard, semisoft and soft. Each has its own
advantages and disadvantages.

There are a few eye-defects which are more amenable
to contact lenses than to glasses. Contact lenses are of great
value in correcting high astigmatism (irregular sight),
keratoconus (cone-shaped cornea) and high anisometropia
(big difference in refractory powers of the two eyes).
Correction of high anisometropia with glasses usually results
into double vision. This difficulty can be overcome with
contact lenses.

Certain defects arising out of the use of glasses can be
overcome with contact lenses. A person can see clearly only
if he sees through the centre of the glass. Perepheral or
paracentral parts of glasses give rise to defects like spherical
aberration, chromatic aberration and coma. Due to this the
person has to contend with a limited field of vision. On the
other hand, since the contact lenses move with the eyes, one
always sees through the centres of the lenses. Hence the
question of above-mentioned defects does not arise.

It is said that contact lenses help to check the increase of eye-defect and the number (of spectacles) becomes steady. However, innumerable cases have been seen where the eye-defect has continued to increase even after the use of contact lenses. In fact, this point needs further elucidation. We know that a visual defect has a tendency to grow along with the growth of the body. In many cases, the defect stops getting worse at around 17 – 18 years of age. It is at this time that the use of contact lenses is resorted to. Thus it is difficult to say whether the eye-numbers have stopped increasing as per the natural course or due to the use of contact lenses.

Experts have drawn attention to some dangers arising out of the use of contact lenses. They are summarised below :

(a) The use of contact lenses is not entirely safe.

(b) If strict hygienic conditions are not maintained during insertion or removal of contact lenses, the eyes may get contaminated with germs and micro-organisms.

(c) The cornea solely depends upon atmospheric oxygen for its nutrition. Contact lenses do not allow atmospheric oxygen to come in contact with cornea. This results into corneal oedema (water-logging).

(d) If proper care is not taken while inserting or removing a contact lens, the cornea might be injured resulting into abrasions and scratches which affect vision.

Thus ophthalmologists have thrown light on probable dangers of contact lens use. Though such complications are rare, one should be aware of them.

The dangers of contact lens use mostly arise if the contact lenses do not fit properly on the eyes. If the lens is prepared without precisely measuring the anterior curvature of the cornea, a number of difficulties like redness and pain in the eyes, corneal swelling, corneal abrasions, decrease in corneal transparency, etc., arise. However, these difficulties do not arise if the lenses are of precise shape, i.e. if their fitting is proper.

A person who opts for contact lenses initially experiences certain difficulties. His eyes water continuously, he experiences dust in his eyes and the rate of blinking increases. Excessive tears sometimes cause displacement of the lens resulting into a red-eye. In some persons, difficulties last about one to four weeks. But if lenses are properly fitted, such difficulties shortly disappear. The extent of such difficulties is much lesser with soft or semisoft lenses.

In conclusion, it can be said that use of contact lenses has its own advantages and disadvantages. However, if the lenses are prepared by an expert and if they are properly fitted, the incidence of difficulties is negligible.

The advantages of their use are obvious. Appearance improves; question of distortion of objects arising out of vision through peripheral parts of glasses does not arise; objects appear to be of their normal size (not larger or smaller as happens with glasses). In some cases, the visual defect stops increasing.

The reader should opt for contact lenses only after giving thought to all aspects of their advantages and disadvantages.

12. GENERAL CARE OF EYES

People, especially those of villages, are not fully conscious about eye-care. Some basic facts about eyes and eye-care have been given below :

(1) **Diet :** Blindness due to vitamin A deficiency is still rampant in villages of our country. In fact, vitamin deficiencies can easily be avoided by regular intake of green leafy vegetables and milk which are easily available in villages.

(2) **General hygiene :** Eyes should be protected from dust and smoke. Eyes should be cleaned twice during the day with simple water or saline.

(3) One should never look directly at the sun. One should be especially careful at the time of a solar eclipse.

(4) If a dust particle enters an eye, do not rub the eye. Dip the eye in a vessel containing pure water and then blink. The dust particle will be washed away.

(5) When there is an epidemic of conjunctivitis, one should try to keep away from such patients. A person suffering from conjunctivitis should be segregated. His clothes and handkerchieves should not be used by others. They should be boiled and washed separately.

(6) One should cultivate habits that would strengthen the eyes and also learn the correct methods of using them.

(7) One should remain alert while bursting crackers or playing games which are likely to hurt eyes.

————

USEFUL THERAPEUTIC MAGNETS AND MAGNETIC APPLIANCES

1. **High Power Magnets** *(Pair)*
   For the treatment of joints and for magnetizing water

2. **Medium Power Magnets** *(Pair)*
   To treat diseases of the chest and the abdomen

3. **Low Power Magnets** *(Pair)*
   For the treatment of small or delicate organs

4. **Very Small Magnets** *(Ten Pieces)*
   To stick for a couple of days on specific points of the skin

5. **Magnetic Spectacles** *(With Pinholes)*
   For the treatment of visual and eye-disorders

6. **Magnetic Wrist Belt**
   To control blood pressure

7. **Magnetic Back Belt** *(in Various sizes)*
   For the treatment of back or abdominal disorders

8. **Magnetic Knee Belt**
   For the treatment of knee-disorders

9. **Magnetic Neck Belt**
   For the treatment of neck-disorders

10. **Magnetic Head Belt**
    For the treatment of headache, insomnia, mental tension, etc.

11. **Magnetic Necklace**
    For the treatment of respiratory disorders

12. **Magnetic Chest Belt**
    To relieve an acute attack of asthma

13. **Magnetic Tonsil Belt**
    For the treatment of tonsillitis, laryngitis, sore throat

14. **Magnetic Pain (Calf) Belt**
    To treat pain/cramps in calf, thigh, arm, forearm

15. **Magnetic Seat**
    To treat piles, menstrual disorders, hydrocele, etc.

Available with

SONA MAGNETS C/o. Dr. Gala

Abbas Building 'A', 1st floor, Near Tilak Market,
Jalbhai Road, Grant Road (East), MUMBAI–400 004.
Phone : 2386 7275, Time : 4 to 7 p.m.

E 27

BE YOUR OWN DOCTOR WITH
MAGNET THERAPY

Are you disillusioned with medicines?
Is your disease such that cannot be cured by medicines?
Are you apprehensive of the adverse side-effects of medicines?
Do you want to actively participate in the process of your recovery?
Do you desire not falling ill at all?
Do you want to prevent old age, i.e., stay young forever?

THEN ADOPT MAGNET THERAPY

Magnet therapy is a simple, harmless and effective mode of treatment. More and more people are turning to Magnet therapy to regain lost health. Magnet therapy is not only good but cheap too since magnets once bought, serve like faithful servants for years, helping to preserve and/or regain health.

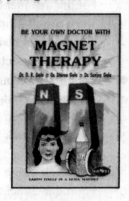

CAUTION

Some confusion prevails regarding the nomenclature of magnetic poles, i.e., which pole of a magnet should be called south and which pole should be called north.

A magnet suspended with a light string, after a while, stabilises in the north-south direction. That surface or pole of the magnet which faces the north direction should be named and labelled 'the north pole' and that surface or pole of the magnet which faces the south must be named and labelled 'the south pole.' This universal convention has been followed throughout this book.

The reader should ensure that the magnets he buys from the market are correctly marked. The north and the south poles of a magnet have mutually opposite properties and effects. Hence, when only one pole of the magnet is to be used, it is imperative that it is the right one. Otherwise, the desired benefits will not accure.

A BOOK NO HEALTH-CONSCIOUS PERSON CAN DO WITHOUT

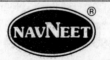

E 3

BACKACHE
PREVENTION AND CURE

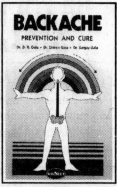

Unless their backs are giving trouble, people take it for granted that their backs are in good shape. They could be wrong. In fact, they often are. Considering the alarming prevalence of backaches, there is a good likehood that the day will soon come when they will end up in a doctor's clinic, pleading for relief from incapacitating back pain.

- If you are an executive, leading a sedentary life
- If you are a worker required to take on sporadic physical tasks
- If you are a pregnant woman
- If you find your back stiff and uncomfortable in the morning
- If you play sports only on week-ends and find on Monday that your back is acting up
- If you have suffered from a backache earlier

THEN YOU ARE A PRIME CANDIDATE FOR BACK PROBLEMS

Don't wait till an attack of backache strikes. Take appropriate steps to prevent it.

Most backaches are caused by weakness or shortness of one or more muscles associated with the back. This book describes a simple 'seven-step test' to assess the efficiency of back muscles. Take this test today and find out how your muscles measure up.

The book also describes simple and effective exercises to strengthen weak muscles. With your back thus reconditioned, you shall be able to thumb your nose at backache—forever!

If backache has already struck, the book will enable you to understand what your doctor says. Besides, it will also suggest what you can do yourself to overpower pain. It will then proceed to show you the way to prevent a recurrence of pain.

IF YOU FEEL CONCERNED FOR YOUR OWN HEALTH AND THAT OF YOUR FAMILY, THIS BOOK IS A MUST FOR YOU.

E 13

GALA PUBLISHERS OFFER
Very useful, low priced health books

1. Be Your Own Doctor with Acupressure
2. Be Your Own Doctor with Foot Reflexology
3. Be Your Own Doctor with Magnet Therapy
4. Nature Cure for Common Diseases
5. Juice-Diet for Perfect Health
6. Efficacy of Fasting
7. Prevent Heart Disease and Prolong Life
8. From Fat to Fit
9. Backache : Prevention and Cure
10. Diabetes, High Blood Pressure, Without Any Fear
11. Panacea on the Earth : Wheat Grass Juice
12. Vision Training Programme
13. Care of the Eyes
14. Incurable Disease? Don't Despair
15. Auto-Urine Therapy
16. Be Your Own Doctor Using REIKI
17. Yoga : Yogasanas and Pranayama for Health
18. Holy Basil Tulsi
19. The Pregnancy and Baby-Care Book
20. Health in Your Hands (Reflexology) : Volume 1
21. Health in Your Hands : Volume 2 (Parts 1–2)
22. Defeat the Dragon
23. Homoeopathy for Common Diseases
24. Acupressure Chart
25. Shivambu Geeta
26. Defeat Depression
27. A Unique Remedy for A Hundread Ailments : Fasting
28. Health Aerobic and Beauty
29. Arthritis ? Try Yogasanas
30. Health at Your Fingertips
31. Our Valued Treasure – Our Children

Where knowledge is wealth™

E 25